T0016938

To:

From:

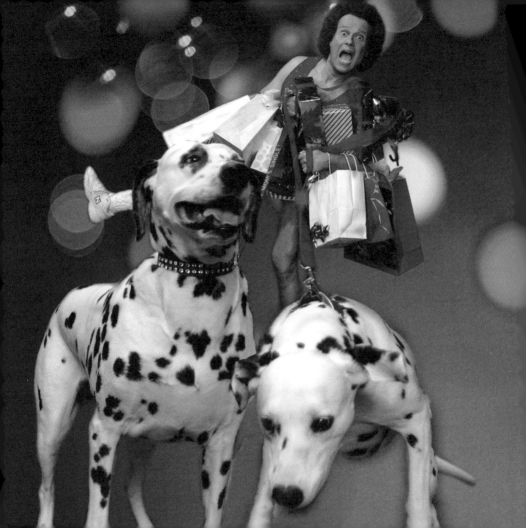

Richard Simmons
12 DAYS OF
Richard Simmons

Penguin Workshop

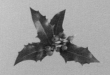

PENGUIN WORKSHOP
An imprint of Penguin Random House LLC, New York

First published in the United States of America by Penguin Workshop,
an imprint of Penguin Random House LLC, New York, 2022

© Jemini LLC

All images not of Richard Simmons are credited to Getty Images.

Visit us online at penguinrandomhouse.com.

Manufactured in China

ISBN 9780593520598   10 9 8 7 6 5 4 3 2 1 TOPL

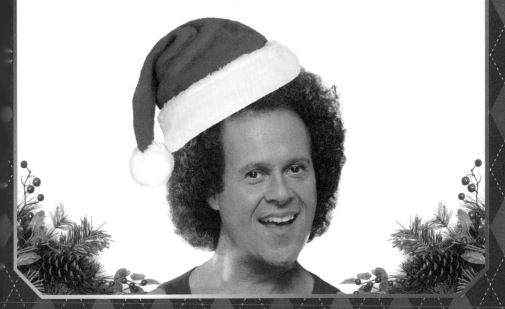

★Richard Simmons

12 DAYS OF
Richard Simmons

Everyone in this world
is somehow connected . . .
so why not just be nice
to everybody.

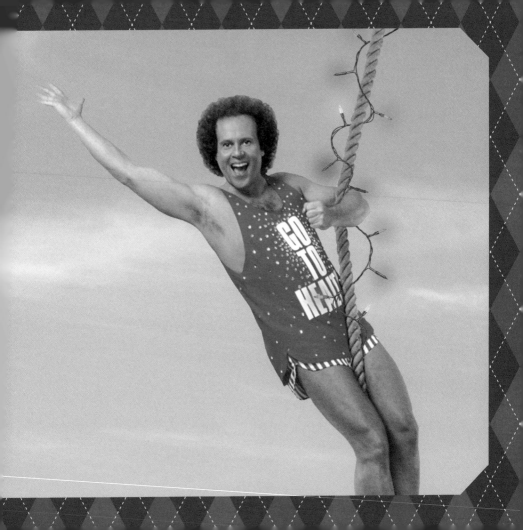

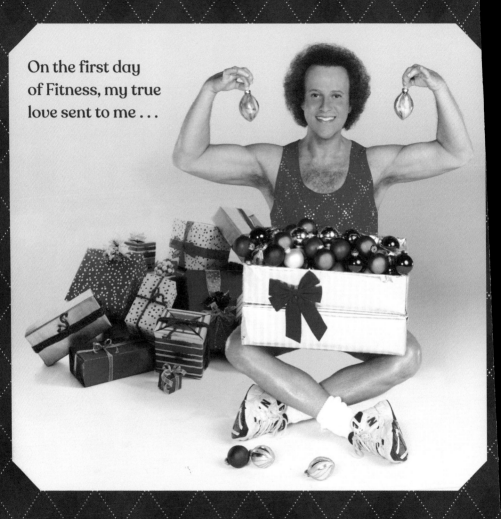

On the first day of Fitness, my true love sent to me . . .

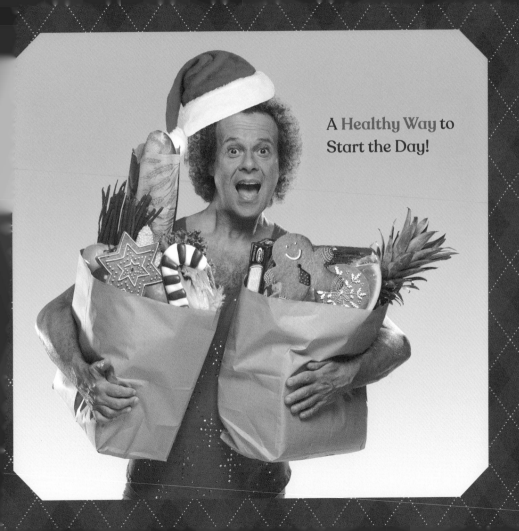

A Healthy Way to
Start the Day!

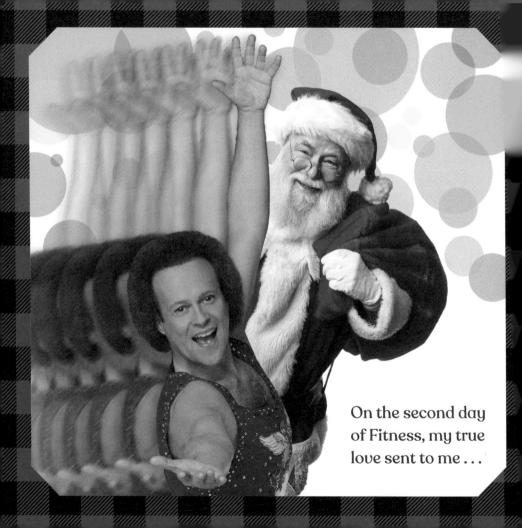

On the second day of Fitness, my true love sent to me . . .

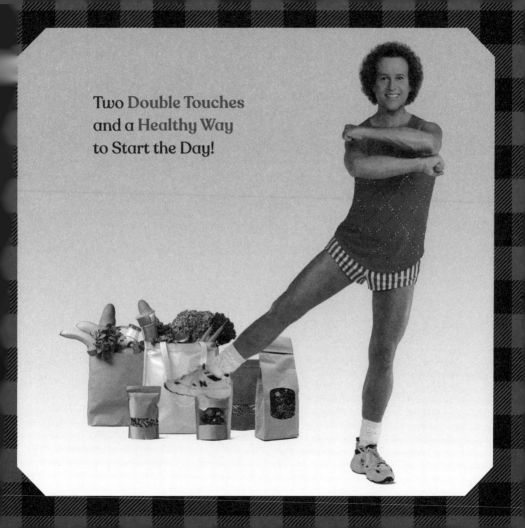

Two Double Touches
and a Healthy Way
to Start the Day!

On the third day
of Fitness, my true
love sent to me . . .

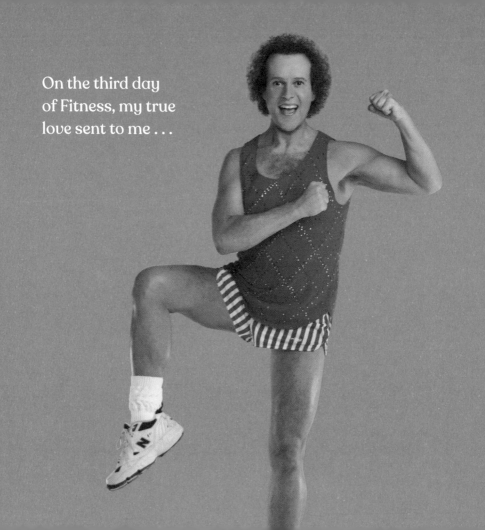

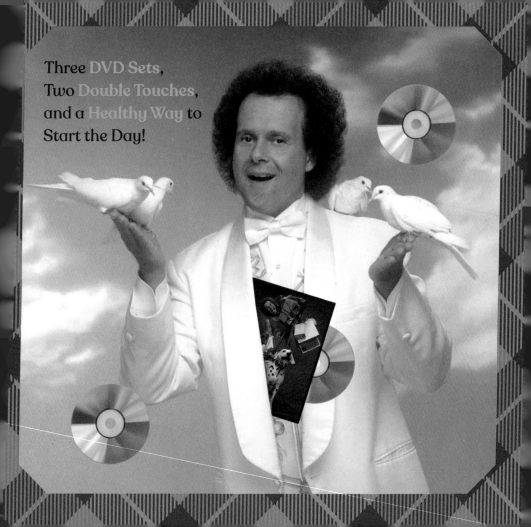

Three DVD Sets, Two Double Touches, and a Healthy Way to Start the Day!

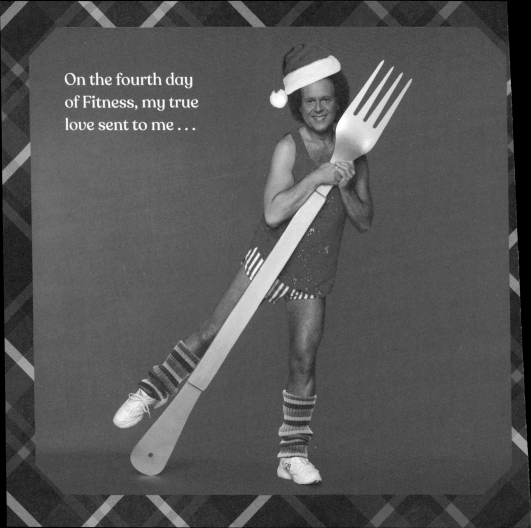

On the fourth day
of Fitness, my true
love sent to me . . .

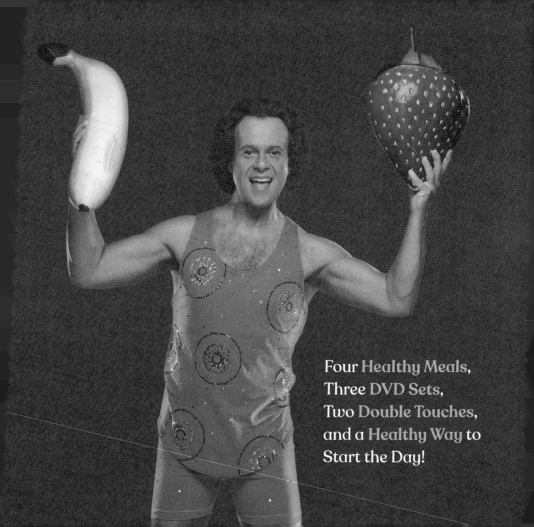

Four **Healthy Meals**,
Three **DVD Sets**,
Two **Double Touches**,
and a **Healthy Way** to
Start the Day!

On the fifth day of Fitness, my true love sent to me . . .

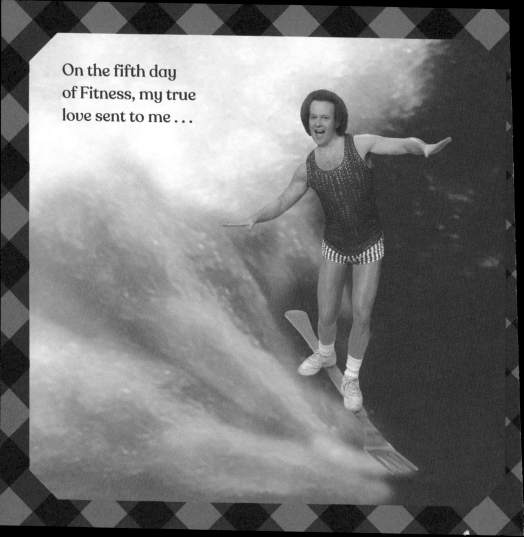

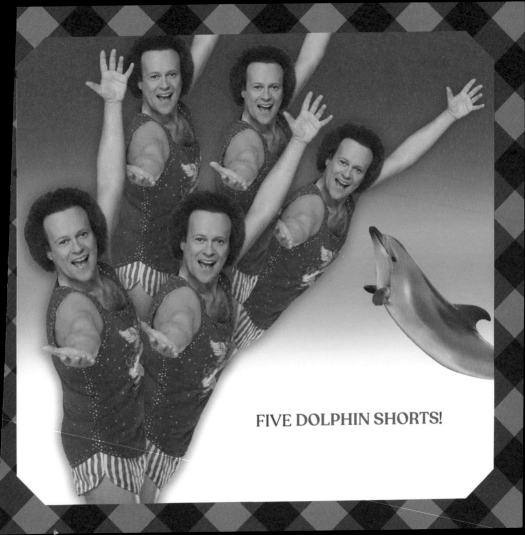

FIVE DOLPHIN SHORTS!

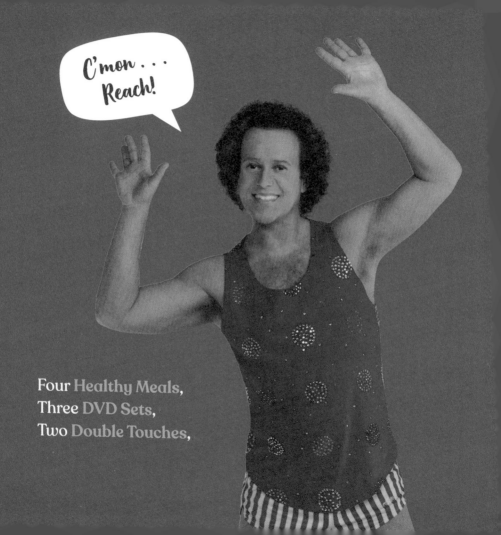

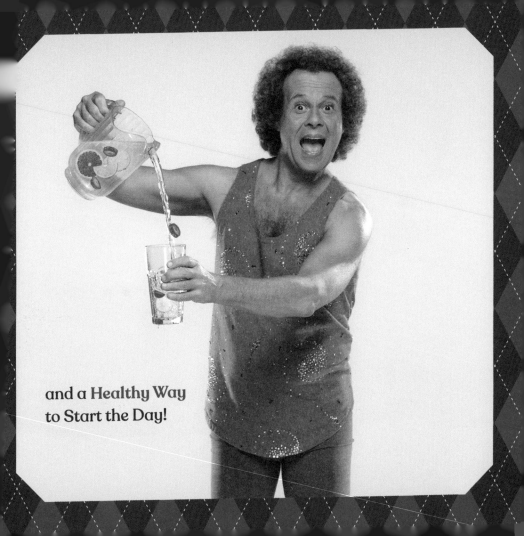

and a Healthy Way
to Start the Day!

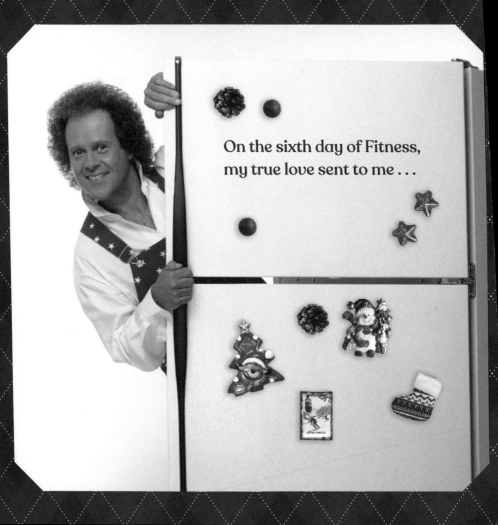

On the sixth day of Fitness,
my true love sent to me . . .

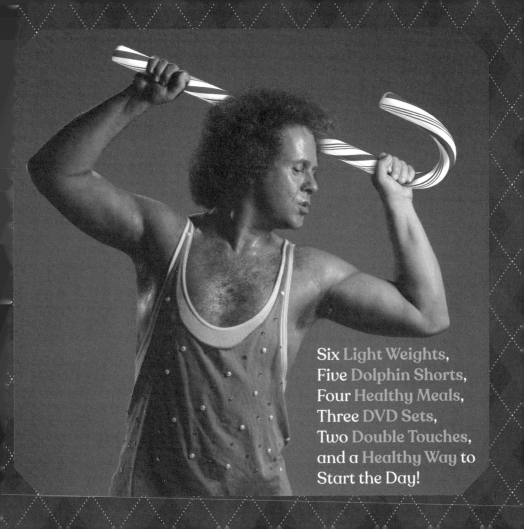

Six Light Weights,
Five Dolphin Shorts,
Four Healthy Meals,
Three DVD Sets,
Two Double Touches,
and a Healthy Way to
Start the Day!

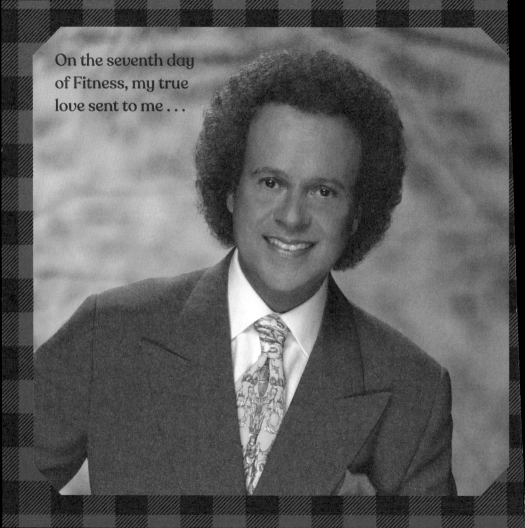

On the seventh day of Fitness, my true love sent to me . . .

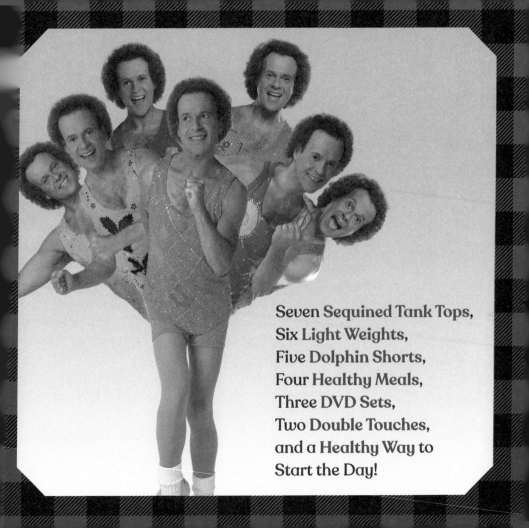

Seven Sequined Tank Tops,
Six Light Weights,
Five Dolphin Shorts,
Four Healthy Meals,
Three DVD Sets,
Two Double Touches,
and a Healthy Way to
Start the Day!

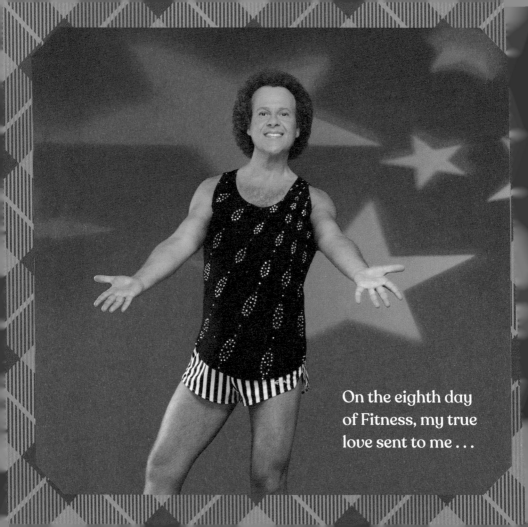

On the eighth day
of Fitness, my true
love sent to me . . .

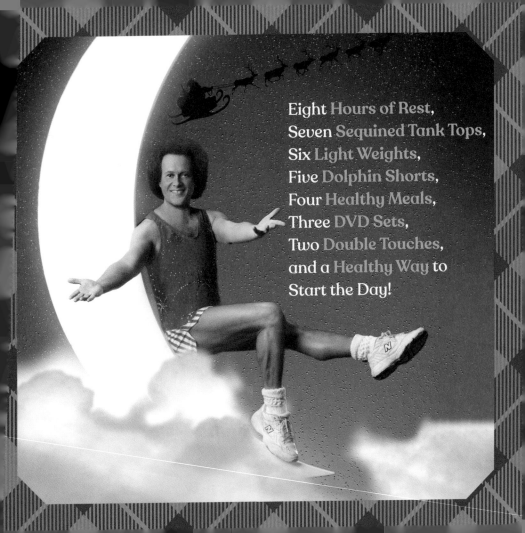

Eight Hours of Rest,
Seven Sequined Tank Tops,
Six Light Weights,
Five Dolphin Shorts,
Four Healthy Meals,
Three DVD Sets,
Two Double Touches,
and a Healthy Way to
Start the Day!

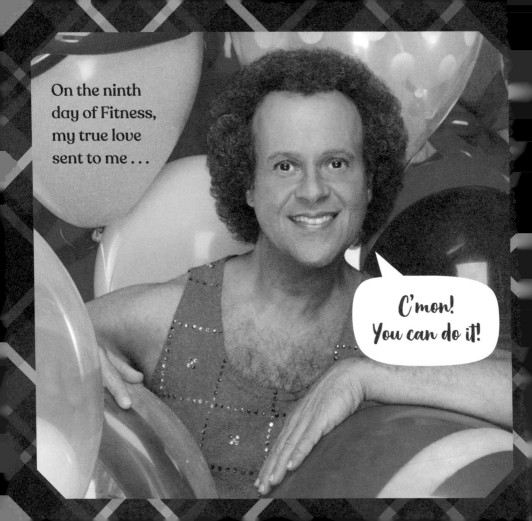

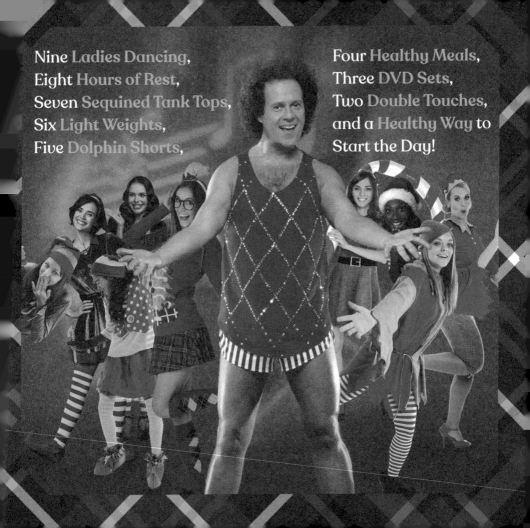

Nine Ladies Dancing,
Eight Hours of Rest,
Seven Sequined Tank Tops
Six Light Weights,
Five Dolphin Shorts,

Four Healthy Meals,
Three DVD Sets,
Two Double Touches,
and a Healthy Way to
Start the Day!

On the tenth day
of Fitness, my true
love sent to me . . .

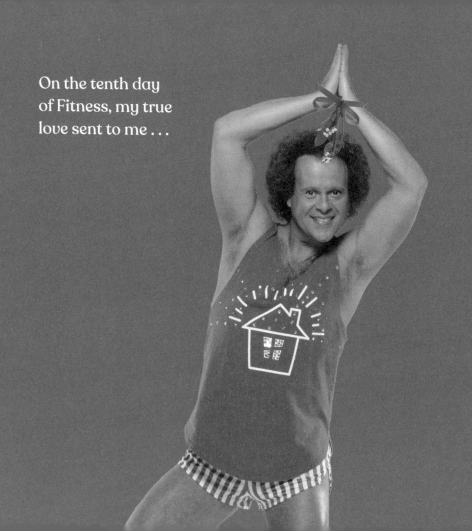

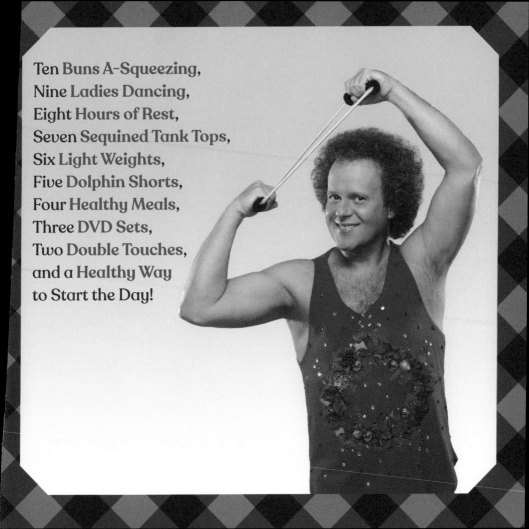

Ten Buns A-Squeezing,
Nine Ladies Dancing,
Eight Hours of Rest,
Seven Sequined Tank Tops,
Six Light Weights,
Five Dolphin Shorts,
Four Healthy Meals,
Three DVD Sets,
Two Double Touches,
and a Healthy Way
to Start the Day!

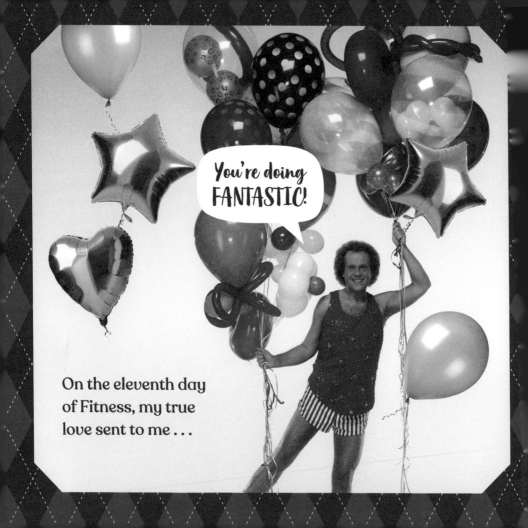

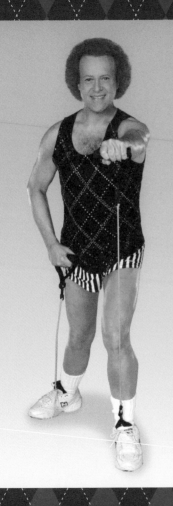

Eleven Lads A-Lunging,
Ten Buns A-Squeezing,
Nine Ladies Dancing,
Eight Hours of Rest,
Seven Sequined Tank Tops,
Six Light Weights,
Five Dolphin Shorts,
Four Healthy Meals,
Three DVD Sets,
Two Double Touches,
and a Healthy Way to
Start the Day!

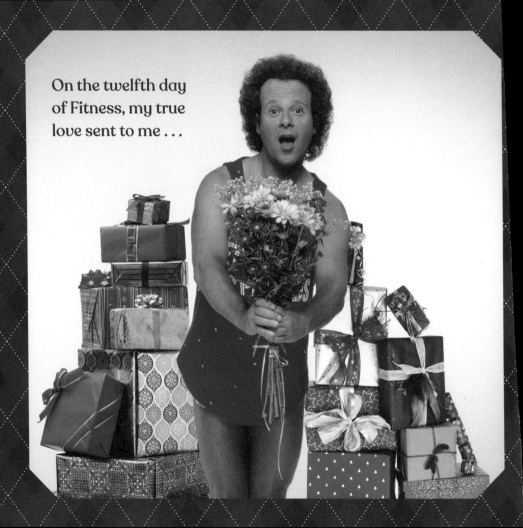

On the twelfth day of Fitness, my true love sent to me . . .

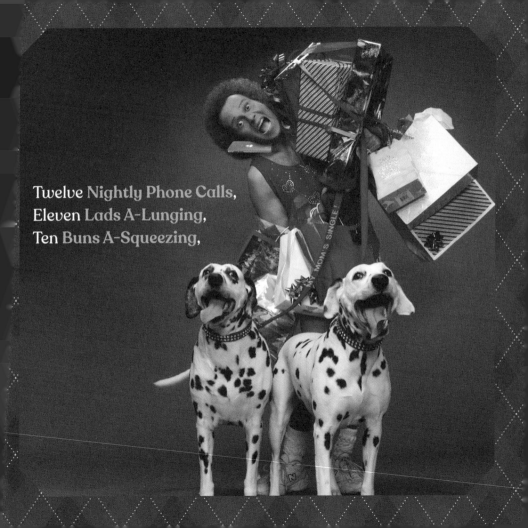

Twelve Nightly Phone Calls,
Eleven Lads A-Lunging,
Ten Buns A-Squeezing,

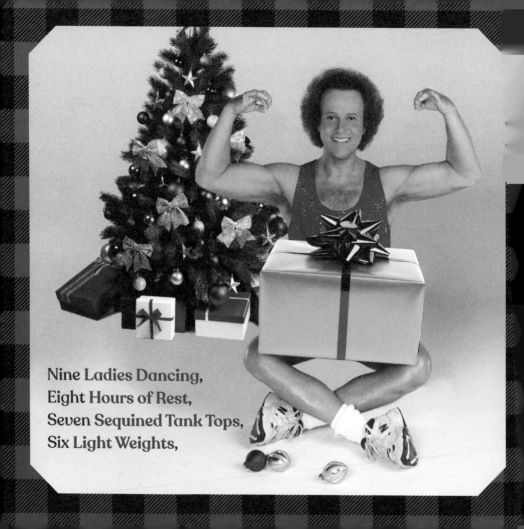

Nine Ladies Dancing,
Eight Hours of Rest,
Seven Sequined Tank Tops,
Six Light Weights,

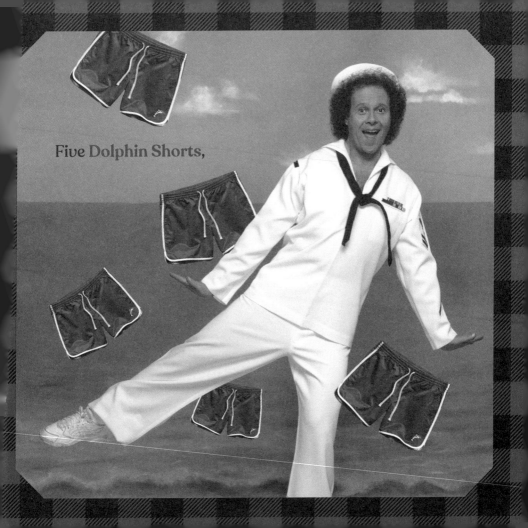

Five Dolphin Shorts,

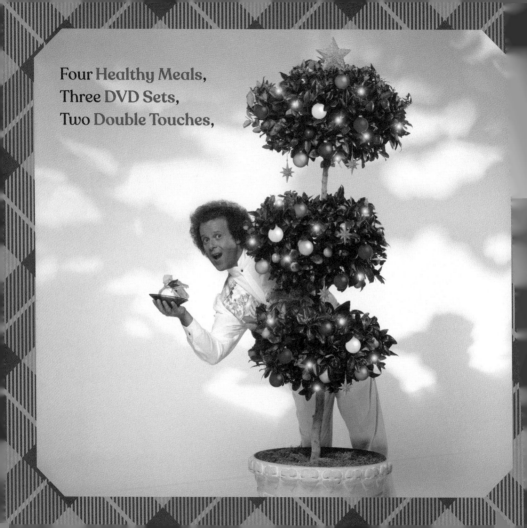

Four **Healthy Meals,**
Three **DVD Sets,**
Two **Double Touches,**

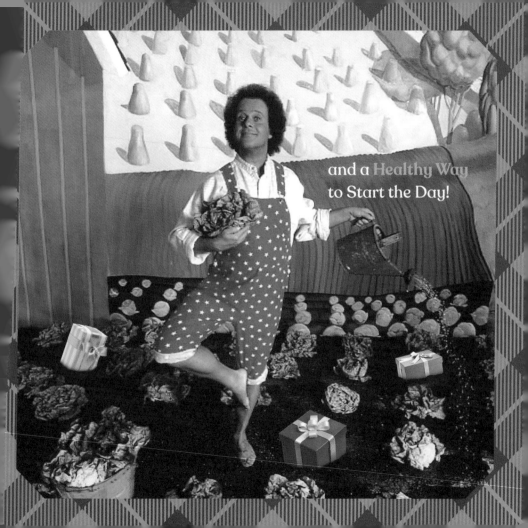

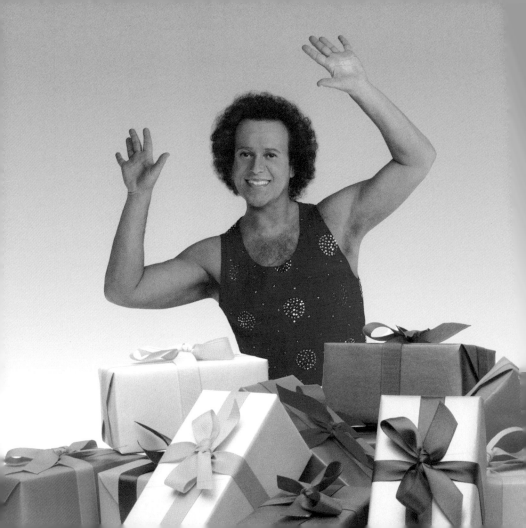

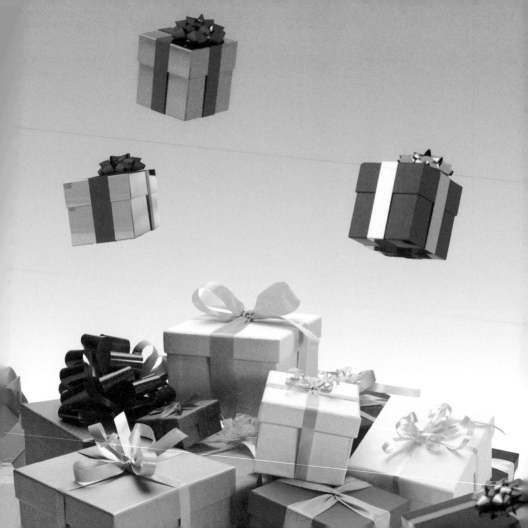

Work hard, take care
of yourself, and
you'll be just fine.

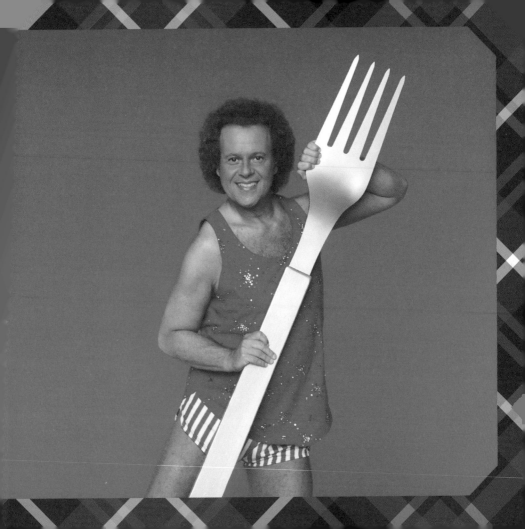

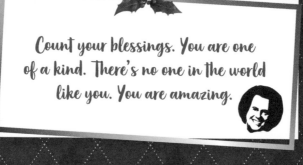

Count your blessings. You are one of a kind. There's no one in the world like you. You are amazing.